Autoimmune Cookbook

Autoimmune All-Day Recipes

All Rights Reserved. No part of this publication may be reproduced in any form or by any means, including scanning, photocopying, or otherwise without prior written permission of the copyright holder. Copyright © 2014

About the Author – Melissa Groves

Melissa passionately believes that eating healthy shouldn't have to mean surviving on steamed vegetables. Her interest in nutrition first began when she was majoring in dance in college. Figuring out ways to make healthy foods taste good became her obsession. She enjoys creating recipes that meet specific dietary needs without sacrificing taste.

She recently left a 15-year career in advertising in NYC to pursue a degree in Nutrition, with the goal of becoming a registered dietitian. She is a 2000 graduate of the Institute for Integrative Nutrition. Her recipes have won national awards.

She now lives on the NH Seacoast, where she is an active part of the local food movement. In addition to scouring the local farmers' markets and cooking, she enjoys running on the beach, hiking, and traveling.

Table of Contents

Why the Autoimmune Protocol?

Foods to Avoid

Chapter 1 – **Breakfast**

Green Piña Colada Smoothie

Triple Berry Smoothie

Zesty Grapefruit Bowl

Tropical Breakfast Salad

Sweet Potato Breakfast Porridge

Chapter 2 – **Lunch**

Chilled Cucumber Avocado Soup

Creamy Butternut Squash Soup

Gingery Carrot Beet Soup

Shrimp "Tacos"

Cucumber "Sushi"

Summer Rolls with Mango Dipping Sauce

Balsamic Beet and Orange Salad

Nicoise Salad

Strawberry Salmon Salad

Chopped Chicken Salad

Chapter 3 – **Dinner**

Shrimp Scampi Spaghetti Squash

Cod with Basil Pesto

Halibut with Olive Tapenade

Coconut Chicken Stirfry

Roasted Chicken with Root Vegetables

Turkey Burgers with Fries

Slow-Cooked Pulled Pork and Cabbage

Slow-Cooked Beef Stew

Shepherd's Pie

Broiled Lamb Chops with Slaw

Chapter 4 – **Snacks**

Red and Green Apple Cinnamon Crisps

Baked Kale Chips

Prosciutto & Melon

Jicama Sticks with Guacamole

Coconut Ice Cream

Why the Autoimmune Protocol?

Every day, dozens of people across the country get diagnosed with one or more autoimmune condition: systemic lupus erythematosus, celiac disease, Graves' disease, rheumatoid arthritis, type 1 diabetes... All these conditions and many more are caused by a dysfunction of the immune system. Normally, the immune system is responsible for fighting off microorganisms such as viruses, bacteria and fungi that would otherwise invade our bodies. However, some people's immune system has difficulty differentiating between self and non-self. Essentially, these people's immune system attacks their own body tissues. Some auto-immune diseases destroy the intestines, while others destroy joints, organs, skin or glands.

Science doesn't know the exact reasons why some people's immune system will attack healthy body tissues. What we do know is that many autoimmune reactions are in fact a response to a trigger: drugs, viruses or bacteria, irritants, food, etc. For example, someone with celiac disease will suffer intestinal damage after eating food that contains gluten (a protein found in wheat, barley and rye). Other people are sensitive to specific vegetables, chemicals or environmental triggers that cause heavy inflammation in their joints. In other words, autoimmune conditions seem to be similar to allergies, but with chronic consequences rather than an immediate reactions such as those seen when people come in contact with allergens. This leads the scientific community to further try to understand the role of inflammation in autoimmunity.

There are strong beliefs that some specific foods are more likely to trigger autoimmune reactions. These foods contain certain toxins, proteins or molecules that cause inflammation and trigger autoimmune reactions. This interesting topic has led to the creation of a very restrictive diet designed to eliminate all the common inflammation-causing "problem foods" from one's diet and reintroduce them one at a time in order to identify the culprit(s). This diet is known as the autoimmune protocol (AIP). The goal of the autoimmune protocol is to allow the person's immune system to rest, lower inflammation levels and allow for recovery. Once inflammation levels are low enough and the gut is healed, the person can start reintroducing foods one by one, carefully monitoring any resulting autoimmune flare-ups. Since the autoimmune protocol is generally pretty boring, most people are excited to reintroduce foods after several weeks.

It is important to *avoid cheating* while on the AIP. A small slip-up could ruin your efforts at trying to figure out which foods are causing your immune system to attack your own body. Healing from the damage done by inflammation is extremely important: chronic inflammation can lead to pain, loss of mobility, organ failure and several other potentially serious complications. Inflammation is the result of the immune system's attempt at eradicating a "threat" (the food you're eating) by launching a generalized inflammation attack all over your tissues and organs. Most people feel significantly better on the AIP and many decide to keep an anti-inflammatory diet for the rest of their lives. The Paleolithic diet is a very popular follow-up to the autoimmune protocol because of its major health benefits on inflammation levels.

How should you reintroduce foods? The key is to start small. Have a bite, then have a large portion of it later the same day. You need to eat enough of it to create a response. If you haven't responded after 4-5 days, chances are that you have no antibodies against that specific food. It can be considered safe and added to your regular diet. If you react to a food, it needs to be banned as it will nearly always trigger your immune system, much like an allergic person will always react to peanuts/shrimp/pollen/etc. Reactions can widely vary in nature, from "brain fog" and lethargy to insomnia, depression and disease flare-ups.

The autoimmune protocol is a very basic diet. It consists of fruits, vegetables and meat. However, not all vegetables are allowed: a specific family of vegetables known as nightshades causes autoimmune reactions in a large amount of people. The nightshade family includes eggplants, tomatoes, peppers (sweet and hot kinds – even chilies and jalapeños), mustard and potatoes. Artificial and no-calorie sweeteners are banned, as are processed foods, vegetable oils, dairy, grains, nuts, seeds, legumes, eggs, dried fruit and alcohol. What you can eat: meat (preferably grass-fed), fish and seafood, around 2 pieces of fruit per day, the occasional use of natural sweeteners (maple syrup, honey) in small amounts, fermented foods, many coconut products including milk, oil and coconut aminos, clarified butter (known as ghee) and non-nightshade veggies. Fats such as olive oil, lard and bacon fat are allowed, as are avocadoes, herbs, green tea and vinegar.

Since sticking to the autoimmune protocol is the key to its success, it is important to gather as much information as possible before starting. Of course, a cookbook containing creative autoimmune-friendly recipes is also a handy addition to your kitchen, as you will soon realize that you can't cook most of your favorite meals. Having such a cookbook can make following AIP guidelines easier as well. You can make AIP meals enjoyable by thinking outside the box and this cookbook is here to accomplish just that: inspire you to create healthy, anti-inflammatory meals that will make you feel truly great.

Foods to Avoid

You will want to avoid:

- Anything pre-packaged, canned or boxed, including frozen entrees and prepared salads or sandwiches. Most pre-packaged foods contain foods to avoid and are heavily processed. Canned or frozen veggies (excluding tomatoes) and pre-packaged baby spinach or lettuce mixes are generally fine
- No-calorie sweeteners and sugar substitutes, including stevia, xylitol and other sugar alcohols, sucralose, aspartame, acesulfame-k
- Added sugar (soda, candy and chocolate are obvious, but sugar is in everything including vinaigrettes and canned vegetables)
- All grains: wheat, barley, rye, rice, quinoa, amaranth, buckwheat, wild rice, oats, kamut, millet, sorghum, etc.
- Dairy, including butter, cheese, milk and yogurt. The *only* exception is cultured ghee (clarified butter, certified free of casein and lactose)
- Alcohol and excess caffeine (green tea is fine)
- Eggs
- Legumes: all dried beans, chickpeas, soy, edamame, hummus, etc. Green and string beans are fine
- Nuts and their oils
- Seeds and their oils: chia, flax, hemp, seed-based spices such as cumin and coriander, mustard, nutmeg, caraway, poppyseed

- Dried fruit and fructose (2 pieces of fresh fruit per day are acceptable)
- Nightshades: potatoes, tomatoes, sweet peppers (green, yellow, red, orange), hot peppers, chilies, eggplant
- Vegetable oils, except olive and coconut

Chapter 1

Breakfast

Green Piña Colada Smoothie

Prep Time: 5 minutes

Cook Time: N/A

Servings: 1

INGREDIENTS

1 cup pineapple

1 cup raw kale or spinach

½ cup coconut water

2 ice cubes

1 Tablespoon coconut oil

1 lime, squeezed (about 2 Tablespoons)

1 teaspoon ground ginger (or 1 inch fresh ginger, peeled)

INSTRUCTIONS

1. Add pineapple, coconut water, ginger, and ice cubes to blender. Blend until smooth.
2. Add the remaining ingredients to the blender and process until smooth.

Triple Berry Smoothie

Prep Time: 5 minutes

Cook Time: N/A

Servings: 1

INGREDIENTS

1 banana, fresh or frozen

½ cup blackberries

½ cup raspberries

½ cup strawberries

½ cup coconut water or filtered water

1 Tablespoon coconut oil

INSTRUCTIONS

1. Add all ingredients to the blender and blend until smooth.

Zesty Grapefruit Bowl

Prep Time: 5 minutes

Cook Time: N/A

Servings: 1

INGREDIENTS

1 pink grapefruit, peeled, sectioned, and chopped

1 avocado, peeled and chopped

½ cup chopped fresh mint

½ Tablespoon apple cider vinegar

½ Tablespoon olive oil

Dash of sea salt

INSTRUCTIONS
1. Combine all ingredients in a bowl.
2. Serve immediately, or chill overnight.

Tropical Breakfast Salad

Prep Time: 10 minutes

Cook Time: N/A

Servings: 1

INGREDIENTS

1 mango, peeled and chopped

1 kiwi, peeled and chopped

¼ cup shredded toasted coconut

1 lime, squeezed (about 2 Tablespoons)

1 Tablespoon coconut oil

½ teaspoon ground cinnamon

½ teaspoon ground ginger

INSTRUCTIONS

1. Combine mango, kiwi, and coconut in a bowl and mix.
2. Combine lime, coconut oil, and spices in a shaker jar or blender and process until combined.
3. Pour dressing over the salad.

Sweet Potato Breakfast Porridge

Prep Time: 10 minutes

Cook Time: 30 minutes

Servings: 2

INGREDIENTS

2 medium sweet potatoes

1 banana, sliced

½ cup coconut milk

¼ cup shredded toasted coconut

½ teaspoon ground cinnamon

½ teaspoon ground ginger

½ teaspoon sea salt

INSTRUCTIONS

1. Peel and chop the sweet potato. Add to a pot of water to cover and bring to a boil. Cook until potatoes are soft, then drain the water and return potatoes to the pot.
2. Add banana coconut milk, coconut oil, ginger, and salt, to the pot and mash with a potato masher.
3. Serve in bowls topped with toasted coconut.

Chapter 2

Lunch

Chilled Cucumber Avocado Soup

Prep Time: 5 minutes

Chill Time: 30 minutes

Servings: 2

INGREDIENTS

2 large English cucumbers

1 ripe avocado, chopped

½ cup fresh cilantro

1 cup filtered water

1 lime, squeezed (about 2 Tablespoons)

1 teaspoon sea salt

INSTRUCTIONS

4. Roughly chop cucumber and add it to a blender with the cilantro and water. Process until smooth.
5. Add the remaining ingredients to the blender and process until smooth.
6. Chill in the refrigerator for at least 30 minutes or until ready to serve.

Creamy Butternut Squash Soup

Prep Time: 10 minutes

Cook Time: 35 minutes

Servings: 4

INGREDIENTS

1 large yellow onion, chopped

1 large butternut squash (or 4 cups chopped)

2 apples, peeled and chopped

2 Tablespoons apple cider vinegar

4 cups water

1 teaspoon ground cinnamon

1 teaspoon ground ginger (or 1-inch fresh ginger, peeled)

1 teaspoon turmeric

1 teaspoon sea salt

INSTRUCTIONS

1. Sauté onions in olive oil in a large stockpot over medium-high heat until translucent.
2. Add squash and sauté about 5 minutes
3. Add apples, vinegar, water, and spices.
4. Cover and bring to a boil.
5. Reduce heat to medium and simmer for approximately 30 minutes, until squash is tender.
6. Puree the soup with a hand blender, or in batches in a blender or food processor.

Gingery Carrot Beet Soup

Prep Time: 10 minutes
Cook Time: 35 minutes
Servings: 4

INGREDIENTS

1 large yellow onion, chopped

3 pounds carrots, chopped

2 large beets, peeled and chopped

1-2 inches fresh ginger, peeled and chopped

2 cups broth (chicken or vegetable)

2 cups water

2 Tablespoons coconut oil

1 teaspoon sea salt

INSTRUCTIONS

1. Sauté onions in coconut oil in a large stockpot over medium-high heat until translucent.
2. Add carrots, beets, and ginger, and sauté about 5 minutes
3. Add broth, water, and spices.
4. Cover and bring to a boil.
5. Reduce heat to medium and simmer for approximately 30 minutes, until vegetables are tender.
6. Puree the soup with a hand blender, or in batches in a blender or food processor.

Shrimp "Tacos"

Prep Time: 10 minutes

Cook Time: 5 minutes

Servings: 2

INGREDIENTS

12 jumbo shrimp, cleaned, with tails off

4 large lettuce leaves

1 avocado, chopped

1 Tablespoon olive oil

1 cup jicama, grated

½ cup fresh cilantro, chopped

1 lime, cut into 4 wedges

Sea salt to taste

INSTRUCTIONS

1. Sauté the shrimp in olive oil until opaque on both sides.
2. Wash the lettuce and pat the leaves dry with paper towels. Put 2 leaves on each of 2 serving plates.
3. Spoon 3 shrimp onto each of the lettuce leaves.
4. Top each with jicama, avocado, and cilantro.
5. Squeeze lime over each lettuce taco and salt to taste.

Cucumber "Sushi"

Prep Time: 20 minutes

Chill Time: 30 minutes

Servings: 2

INGREDIENTS

4 sheets of nori

2 avocadoes, mashed

8 ounces smoked salmon

1 large cucumber

1 large carrot

½ cup watercress (optional)

Daikon radish (optional)

INSTRUCTIONS

1. Cut cucumber, carrot, and daikon into long thin strips.
2. Cut salmon into long thin strips.
3. Place nori sheet flat on a hard surface, with the shiny side facing down.
4. Spread 1/4 of the mashed avocado evenly over the nori.
5. Place 1/4 of the salmon and vegetables in a long strip in the middle of the piece of nori.
6. Roll the nori tightly from one end to the other, using the avocado to help it "stick."
7. Repeat with the other 3 sheets.
8. Chill for about 30 minutes.
9. Cut the rolls into pieces with a sharp knife and serve.

Summer Rolls with Mango Dipping Sauce

Prep Time: 15 minutes

Cook Time: N/A

Servings: 2

INGREDIENTS

4 large lettuce leaves

8 ounces cooked, shredded chicken

1 medium cucumber, peeled

¼ cup fresh cilantro

¼ cup fresh mint

¼ cup fresh basil

1 mango, peeled and chopped

2 Tablespoons apple cider vinegar

2 Tablespoons filtered water

1 Tablespoon olive oil

1 teaspoon ground ginger

½ teaspoon sea salt

INSTRUCTIONS

1. Blend the mango, vinegar, water, oil, ginger, and salt in a blender until smooth. Serve in small bowls for dipping.
2. Wash the lettuce and pat the leaves dry with paper towels. Put 2 leaves on each of 2 serving plates.
3. Divide the chicken, cucumber, and herbs between each of the 4 lettuce leaves.

4. Wrap each roll like a burrito, rolling one inch of the top down and one inch of the bottom up. Then roll from left to right.
5. Serve with mango dipping sauce.

Nicoise Salad

Prep Time: 15 minutes

Cook Time: 5 minutes

Servings: 2

INGREDIENTS

2 cans albacore tuna in water

2 cups Boston lettuce

1 small red onion, thinly sliced

1 cup radishes, sliced

1 cup green string beans

¼ cup kalamata olives

2 Tablespoons capers

2 Tablespoons olive oil

2 Tablespoons lemon juice

½ teaspoon dried thyme

½ teaspoon dried basil

½ teaspoon dried oregano

Sea salt to taste

INSTRUCTIONS

1. Trim green beans and steam in about 1/2 inch of water until bright green. Instantly immerse beans in a bowl of ice water.
2. Wash, dry, and tear the lettuce into bite-sized pieces. Divide between 2 serving plates.
3. Arrange the green beans, onion, radishes, olives, and tuna on the beds of lettuce.

4. In a separate bowl, whisk the oil, lemon juice, and spices.
5. Pour the dressing over the salads and top with capers. Add salt to taste.

Strawberry Salmon Salad

Prep Time: 10 minutes

Cook Time: 10 minutes

Servings: 2

INGREDIENTS

12 ounces wild salmon fillets, cut into 2 portions

2 cups mixed salad greens

1 cup strawberries, sliced

1 avocado, peeled and cut into ½-inch cubes

2 Tablespoons olive oil

2 Tablespoons unsweetened balsamic vinegar

1 Tablespoon lemon juice

Sea salt to taste

INSTRUCTIONS

1. Place salmon in a deep-sided sauté pan. Add 1/2-inch water and lemon juice to the pan. Cover and cook over medium high until fish is cooked through (8-10 minutes depending on thickness).
2. Divide the salad greens between 2 serving plates.
3. Arrange salmon, strawberries, and avocado on the lettuce.
4. In a bowl, whisk the oil and vinegar with the salt.
5. Pour the dressing over the salads.

Chopped Chicken Salad

Prep Time: 10 minutes

Cook Time: N/A

Servings: 2

INGREDIENTS

1 package shredded cabbage mix (or 2 cups fresh shredded cabbage)

2 cups chopped cooked chicken breasts

4 pieces of AIP-approved bacon, chopped

2 apples, chopped

1 avocado, peeled and cut into ½-inch cubes

2 Tablespoons olive oil

2 Tablespoons apple cider vinegar

1 teaspoon dried tarragon (optional)

Sea salt to taste

INSTRUCTIONS

1. Divide the cabbage between 2 serving plates.
2. Toss chicken, apples, and avocados in a bowl, then divide between the serving plates.
3. In a bowl, whisk the oil and vinegar with the tarragon and salt.
4. Pour the dressing over the salads.
5. Crumble the bacon on top of the salads.

Chapter 3

Dinner

Shrimp Scampi Spaghetti Squash

Prep Time: 5 minutes

Cook Time: 30 minutes

Servings: 2

INGREDIENTS

1 large spaghetti squash

½ pound shrimp, cleaned, with tails on

4 cloves garlic, minced

3 Tablespoons olive oil, plus 1 teaspoon

½ cup fresh parsley, chopped

1 teaspoon sea salt

INSTRUCTIONS

1. Preheat oven to 400 °F.
2. Cut spaghetti squash in half lengthwise, scoop out the seeds, and place cut-side down on a cookie sheet lightly coated with 1 teaspoon of olive oil. Pierce the skin several times with a fork.
3. Bake spaghetti squash for approximately 30 minutes, until a fork goes through the skin easily.
4. While the squash bakes, sauté the garlic in 2 Tablespoons of olive oil for 1 minute.
5. Add the shrimp to the sauté pan and cook until opaque and pink. Set aside.
6. When the spaghetti squash is done and cool enough to handle, scrape out the strands with a fork into a large bowl (you may want to hold the squash using an oven mitt while you do this).

7. Toss the spaghetti squash strands with the remaining 1 tablespoon of olive oil, the parsley, and the sea salt.
8. Serve spaghetti on plates topped with the sautéed shrimp mixture.

Cod with Basil Pesto

Prep Time: 10 minutes

Cook Time: 20 minutes

Servings: 4

INGREDIENTS

1 pound fresh cod fillets

2 cups fresh basil

¼ cup unsweetened shredded coconut

1 lemon, juiced (about 2 Tablespoons)

¼ cup olive oil, plus 1 Tablespoon

1 clove garlic

1 teaspoon sea salt

Lemon wedges for garnish

INSTRUCTIONS

1. Preheat oven to 400 °F.
2. Lightly coat a baking sheet with part of the 1 Tablespoon of oil. Place the fish on the pan and pour the remainder of the 1 Tablespoon of oil over the fish.
3. Bake for 20 minutes, until opaque.
4. While fish is baking, combine basil, coconut, lemon juice, olive oil, garlic, and salt in a food processor and process 30-45 seconds, until combined but still coarse.
5. Serve cod topped with pesto.

Serve with a green vegetable, such as roasted asparagus.

Halibut with Olive Tapenade

Prep Time: 10 minutes

Cook Time: 20 minutes

Servings: 4

INGREDIENTS

1 pound fresh halibut fillets

1 jar kalamata olives, drained

1 jar green olives (without pimentos), drained

¼ cup olive oil, plus 1 Tablespoon

1 Tablespoon lemon juice

1 clove garlic

½ teaspoon sea salt

INSTRUCTIONS

1. Preheat oven to 400 °F.
2. Lightly coat a baking sheet with part of the 1 Tablespoon of oil. Place the fish on the pan and pour the remainder of the 1 Tablespoon of oil over the fish.
3. Bake for 20-30 minutes, until opaque.
4. While fish is baking, combine olives, olive oil, lemon juice, garlic, and salt in a food processor and process 30-45 seconds, until coarsely chopped.
5. Serve halibut topped with tapenade.

Serve with a green vegetable, such as sautéed spinach.

Coconut Chicken Stir Fry

Prep Time: 20 minutes

Cook Time: 20 minutes

Servings: 4

INGREDIENTS

1 pound chicken meat, cut into 1-inch chunks

1 yellow onion, sliced

1 pound broccoli, chopped

4 Tablespoons coconut oil

4 cloves garlic, chopped

1 Tablespoon grated ginger

1 orange

1 teaspoon sea salt

INSTRUCTIONS

1. Sauté onions in coconut oil in a deep sauté pan or wok for about 3 minutes, or until translucent.
2. Add the chicken and cook, stirring frequently, until lightly browned.
3. Add the broccoli and continue to sauté for a few minutes.
4. In a separate bowl, mix the juice from 1 orange, the garlic, ginger, and salt, and whisk until blended.
5. Pour the sauce over the chicken and broccoli and cover until the broccoli is tender.

Roasted Chicken with Root Vegetables

Prep Time: 15 minutes

Cook Time: 1 hour

Servings: 4

INGREDIENTS

4 large bone-in, skin-on chicken breast halves

6 Tablespoons olive oil

3 Tablespoons apple cider vinegar

1 yellow onion, quartered

4 parsnips, peeled and chopped

2 stalks celery, sliced

2 cups baby carrots

2 cups mushrooms, halved

4 cloves garlic, minced

2 Tablespoons fresh rosemary

1 teaspoon sea salt

INSTRUCTIONS

1. Preheat oven to 400 °F.
2. In a large skillet, brown chicken in 1 Tablespoon of the oil for about 8 minutes per side.
3. In a large roasting pan, toss the vegetables with 2 Tablespoons of the oil.
4. In a separate bowl, mix the apple cider vinegar with the remaining 3 Tablespoons of oil, garlic, salt, and rosemary.

5. Lay the browned chicken breasts on top of the vegetables. Pour the sauce over the chicken and vegetables.
6. Bake for 35-40 minutes until chicken is cooked through and vegetables are tender.

Turkey Burgers with Fries

Prep Time: 15 minutes

Cook Time: 30 minutes

Servings: 4

INGREDIENTS

4 medium sweet potatoes

3 Tablespoons olive oil

1 pound ground turkey

1 red onion, diced

½ cup fresh parsley

2 cloves garlic, minced

2 teaspoons sea salt

½ teaspoon cinnamon

INSTRUCTIONS

1. Preheat the oven to 450 °F.
2. Peel sweet potatoes and cut into 1/2-inch sticks.
3. Toss sweet potatoes in a bowl with olive oil, 1 teaspoon of salt, and cinnamon.
4. Bake in a single layer on a baking sheet for about 25-30 minutes, turning once.
5. While the fries are cooking, mix turkey, onion, parsley, garlic, and 1 teaspoon salt together and form into 4 large patties.
6. Grill on an outdoor grill or pan fry for 7 minutes per side

Slow-Cooked Pulled Pork and Cabbage

Prep Time: 10 minutes

Cook Time: 8-10 hours

Servings: 6

INGREDIENTS

2 pounds pork roast

1 large onion, sliced

4 apples, peeled, cored, and sliced

4 cups red cabbage, coarsely shredded

½ cup water

2 Tablespoons apple cider vinegar

1 teaspoon cinnamon

1 teaspoon sea salt

INSTRUCTIONS

1. Add water, apples, cabbage, onion, and vinegar to slow cooker and stir to combine.
2. Rub salt on the roast, then add it to the crockpot.
3. Cook for 8-10 hours on low.
4. Before serving, shred the pork using 2 forks.
5. Scoop the cabbage-apple mixture onto plates and top with the pulled pork

Slow-Cooked Beef Stew

Prep Time: 15 minutes

Cook Time: 8 hours

Servings: 6

INGREDIENTS

3 pounds beef stew meat

1 yellow onion

4 carrots

2 sweet potatoes, peeled

2 parsnips, peeled

2 turnips, peeled

2 cloves of garlic, minced

2 cups beef broth

1 bay leaf

1 teaspoon thyme

1 teaspoon sea salt

INSTRUCTIONS

1. Add the broth to a slow cooker.
2. Chop the beef into 1-inch chunks (if not already pre-cut) and add to the slow cooker.
3. Add the spices and salt to the slow cooker.
4. Chop the vegetables into 1/2- to 1-inch pieces and add to the slow cooker.
5. Cover and cook on low heat for at least 8 hours.

Shepherd's Pie

Prep Time: 15 minutes

Cook Time: 1 hour and 20 minutes

Servings: 4

INGREDIENTS

2 pounds ground beef

1 onion, chopped

2 stalks of celery, chopped

2 carrots, peeled and chopped

1 cup mushrooms, chopped

4 garlic cloves, minced

1 Tablespoon rosemary

1 head cauliflower

2 Tablespoons olive oil

1 teaspoon sea salt

INSTRUCTIONS

1. Brown the meat with the onion, celery, carrots, mushrooms, and garlic in a large stockpot. Cook until meat is fully cooked, about 15-20 minutes
2. In another stockpot, steam cauliflower for about 20 minutes.
3. Preheat oven to 400 °F.
4. Drain the cauliflower and return it to the pot. Mash it with a potato masher. Mix in the olive oil and sea salt.
5. Transfer the beef mixture to a large casserole pan and pat down with a spatula.

6. Spread the mashed cauliflower over the top of the meat.
7. Bake for 40 minutes, until cauliflower starts to brown.

Broiled Lamb Chops with Slaw

Prep Time: 2 minutes

Cook Time: 12 minutes

Servings: 4

INGREDIENTS

4 lamb chops

4 garlic cloves, minced

2 Tablespoons fresh rosemary

2 Tablespoons olive oil

1 teaspoon sea salt

2 large beets, peeled

4 large carrots, peeled

1 apple

2 Tablespoons apple cider vinegar

INSTRUCTIONS

1. In a bowl, rub chops with olive oil, salt, garlic, and rosemary.
2. Broil for 10-12 minutes (until medium rare)
3. Grate the carrots, beets, and apple and place in a large bowl. Toss with the vinegar.
4. Serve the slaw alongside the lamb.

Chapter 4

Snacks

Red and Green Apple Cinnamon Crisps

Prep Time: 5 minutes

Cook Time: 2 hours

Servings: 4

INGREDIENTS

2 Granny Smith apples

2 red apples (McIntosh or other)

1 teaspoon cinnamon

½ teaspoon sea salt

INSTRUCTIONS

1. Preheat oven to 200 °F.
2. Line 2 baking sheets with parchment paper.
3. Slice the apples thinly into rounds or half-rounds.
4. Place the apples in a single layer on the baking sheets, and sprinkle with cinnamon and salt.
5. Bake for 1 hour.
6. Take the chips out and turn them over. Bake for one more hour until fully done.

Baked Kale Chips

Prep Time: 10 minutes

Cook Time: 30 minutes

Servings: 2

INGREDIENTS

1 large bunch of kale

1 Tablespoon olive oil

½ teaspoon onion powder

½ teaspoon garlic powder

1 teaspoon sea salt

INSTRUCTIONS

1. Preheat oven to 300 °F.
2. Line 2 baking sheets with parchment paper.
3. Remove stems from kale and tear it into pieces. Place the kale into a large bowl.
4. Add the olive oil, and "massage" it into the kale with your hands.
5. Spread the kale evenly between the 2 baking sheets. Sprinkle with the spices.
6. Bake for 15 minutes, then rotate the pans, placing the top pan on the bottom and the bottom pan on the top.
7. Bake for another 15 minutes.

Prosciutto & Melon

Prep Time: 5 minutes

Cook Time: N/A

Servings: 4

INGREDIENTS

½ cantaloupe (or honeydew melon)

6 ounces thinly sliced prosciutto

1 Tablespoon fresh mint leaves, finely chopped

1 Tablespoon apple cider vinegar

½ teaspoon sea salt

INSTRUCTIONS

1. Scoop the seeds out of the melon, if necessary, and trim off the skin.
2. Slice the melon into 6 wedges, lengthwise, and then cut each in half crosswise. (You should have 12 pieces.)
3. Place the melon in a bowl and toss with the mint, vinegar, and salt.
4. Slice the prosciutto into 1-2" wide strips, lengthwise. You should have 12 equal portions.
5. Wrap the prosciutto around each piece of melon and serve on a platter.

Jicama Sticks with Guacamole

Prep Time: 10 minutes

Cook Time: N/A

Servings: 4

INGREDIENTS

1 large jicama*

3 avocados

½ red onion, diced

½ cup cilantro, chopped

1 Tablespoon lime juice

1 teaspoon sea salt

INSTRUCTIONS
1. Peel the jicama. Slice it into French-fry-like sticks.
2. Remove the avocado flesh from the skin and mash in a bowl with the onion and cilantro
3. Place the melon in a bowl and toss with the mint, vinegar, and salt.
4. Slice the prosciutto into 1-2" wide strips, lengthwise. You should have 12 equal portions.
5. Wrap the prosciutto around each piece of melon and serve on a platter.

*This is also good with celery sticks or cucumber spears.

Coconut Ice Cream

Prep Time: 10 minutes
Chill Time: 8 hours
Servings: 4

INGREDIENTS

2 cans full-fat coconut milk, refrigerated
1 banana, frozen
2 dates, pitted (optional)
4 ice cubes
½ teaspoon cinnamon

INSTRUCTIONS

1. Take the coconut milk out of the refrigerator. Flip cans over and open from the bottom. Pour off the liquid into a separate bowl.
2. Add the thick coconut "cream" from the cans to a blender.
3. Add the frozen banana, the cinnamon, the ice, and the dates (if using)*
4. Blend until thick and creamy.
5. Eat immediately or place in the freezer for 15-30 minutes for a harder texture.

*If using an ice cream maker, omit the ice and pour the mixture into the ice cream maker and follow the instructions for your machine.

Printed in Great Britain
by Amazon